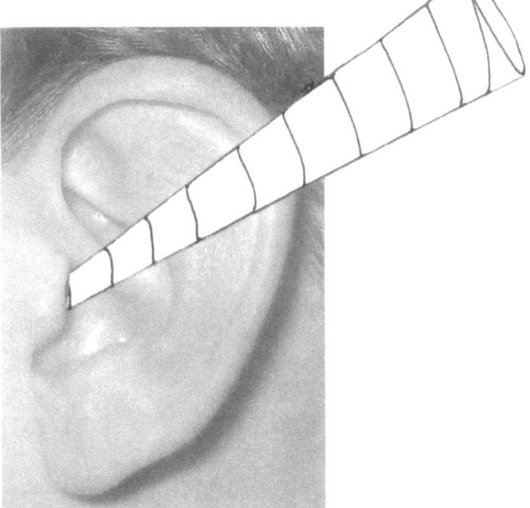

Ear Candler's Manual

Pamper Your Ears with Fire!

Penny Rich

Library of Congress Control Number:		2011960332
ISBN:	Hardcover	978-1-4653-9434-7
	Softcover	978-1-4653-9433-0
	Ebook	978-1-4653-9435-4

This book was printed in the United States of America.

First Printing (Paperback) - July 1989
Second Printing (Paperback) - September 2004
Third Printing (Paperback) -June 2010
Limited Editions

First Edition (Hardcover)—November 2011

To order additional copies of this book, contact:
Xlibris Corporation
1-888-795-4274
www.Xlibris.com
Orders@Xlibris.com
101635

Contents

Dedication...7
Acknowledgments 11
For Your Perusal...13
Important Message About Yeast Infestation............................15
Introduction 17

Chapter I-In the Beginning 19
    Treating the Outer Ear Canal 19
    Balance and Hearing..20
    Who Needs Ear Candling?..21
    Hearing Loss Problems 22
    Serious Ear Infections and How to Avoid Them 22
    Beginning Stages of Hearing Loss.......................................23
    Frequently Asked Questions 24
    Where Does Candida Come From? 24
    How I Became a Certified Ear Coneologist 25
    A Leap of Faith 29
    A Change of Plan 30
    What Did the Doctor Say? 31
    How Does the Ear Cone Work?..31
    Medical vs. Holistic:...33
    How Medical Physicians Feel about Ear Coning....................33
    Vertigo, Dizziness, and Balance Disorders 33
    Drugs That Can Damage the Ear..35
    Ear Coning and How it Benefits Cocaine
        and Other Substance Users 35
    The Pioneer Who Met the Challenge 36
    The Ear and Its Vital Points..36

Chapter II-Purpose of ICEC... 38

    Institute of Certified Ear Candler's 38

    The Ear Candling Procedure 39

    What to Look Forward To..40

    The Human Ear's Mastoid Process..................................43

    Favorable Benefits of Ear Coning 43

    The Ear Has No Natural Process of Elimination 43

    A Special Kodak Moment..44

    The Cover-Up 45

Chapter III-Facts About Ear Wax.. 46

    Ear Wax (Cerumen) Blockage 46

    Water-Related Infections 47

    What Happened in Ketchum, Idaho?..............................50

    The Most Important Final Step 50

    Proper Cleanup Is Essential! 51

    How Much Should Ear Coning Treatment Cost? 52

    When NOT to Treat Ears Holistically 52

    That Strip of Candle Wax...52

    Precautious Measure 53

    The Best Quality Ear Cone...53

    Pure Beeswax vs. Paraffin 53

    The Paraffin Candle 53

    What Is Ear Tinnitus? 53

Chapter IV-Parts of the Human Ear 57

    The External Ear...57

    The Outer Ear..57

    The Middle Ear...58

    The Inner Ear 58

    The Mastoid Process 59

Chapter V-Our First Grads—July 2000 64

The QUESTIONS 65

    The External Ear...65

    The Outer Ear..65

    The Middle Ear...65

The Inner Ear 66
Infections of the Outer Ear Canal...66
Hearing Loss...66
Description of the ICEC Distant Learning Course 67
BEST QUALITY EAR CONES 68

About the Author 69

The ANSWERS..73
Tools of the Trade 77
Important Tips Re: Cleanup Process 77
The Ear Candler's Disclaimer Form......................................78
Other Mind-Body-Spirit Books 79
By Penny Rich...79

Dedication

This book is dedicated to my exquisite mentor, Michael F.
To God in whom I put my trust
To all practitioners of holistic modalities who will find it
to be an invaluable and practical tool.

And to the Media:

Thank you, Gay Yee (former reporter with KCAL-9 News),
for your holistic insight that opened doors to the rejuvenation
of ear coning, and another opportunity to help others.
Thank you, Dave Gonzales (KCAL 9 News Anchor)
for a story well told . . . . as always.

*It was never intended that life be a struggle.
It is but a challenge in an arena wherein the
Light of Experience provides opportunities to
attain spiritual perfection in our quest to
seek and find our highest good.*

—Penny Rich

Acknowledgments

I am incredibly grateful to the many trusting individuals (clients and friends) who believed in what I do as a holistic practitioner.

With special thanks to the woman from India who turned on my light to the joy of this discovery.

The fond memory of my daddy to whom I am forever grateful for the legacy of creative writing.

Thanks to my mother, Laurriet, for teaching me the lesson of patience.

Special thanks to one of my dearest friends over the years, the former California Congresswoman, Diane E. Watson, PhD, for her political influence in making holistic services a recognized and accepted approach to holistic modalities for those of us who would prefer alternatives to conventional medicine.

For Your Perusal

There are very few professionally trained and qualified holistic practitioners who are dedicated to the modality of ear coneology. But those aware of the potential to be of service to others under the astute supervision of a certified technician are best suited to perform in a field that dates back generations in the care and maintenance of the outer ear canal with skills that enhance a metaphysical approach that captures the essence of a very practical and effective alternative method.

Any certified practitioner with knowledge of more than one health care modality such as counseling, herbalist, or any therapeutic holistic practice will find ear coning a delightful way to expand the opportunity to help others; is encouraged to utilize both ear coning and the foot detoxification system offered through the only school of its kind in the United States, the *Institute of Certified Ear Candler's.* Whether it's for use in a private setting or a professional atmosphere we welcome you to explore the concept and take advantage of the expertise provided through years of experience.

The only tool we can't provide is the ability to concentrate and to assist you in keeping your eyes on the flame, as well as being professional when working with your clients. All this treatment requires is a "ton of patience, and a good attitude.

The time it takes to do an ear candling treatment (almost two hours) goes by swiftly when you love people and find pleasure in what you're doing.

Important Message About Yeast Infestation

Definition of Candidiasis
Monilia Albicans: Yeast

Candida albicans are small oval microorganisms known to cause the thriving growth of parasites and other fungi that invade the body causing illness and disease. This (normal) yeast infestation may also inhibit the gastrointestinal tract and may only be kept under control by the Acidophilus bacteria, a natural culture known as *Lactobacillus Acidophilus* grown in skim milk "whey" that are alive with millions of hardy viable organisms.

Beginning in the intestinal track, they start to invade the entire body if not treated, causing such problems as colds and such maladies as *Bell's palsy, Meniere's disease (a balance disorder), and even Alzheimer's disease and dementia, disabling the ability to concentrate and to suffer the loss of reasoning power so commonly found in elderly people. This also includes manic depression, mood swings, and migraine headaches. Later stages present abnormal fatigue, irritability, and constant tiredness due to the toxicity of yeast-infested microorganisms.

Colonies may progress to the external part of the anus where a moist membrane invites them to bud and thrive.

Bell's palsy may indeed be caused by yeast-infested jaw muscles that are eventually paralyzed causing the facial muscles to draw inward and look distorted for weeks.

Introduction

Prior to January 2000, there were no registered certification programs available to become trained ear coneologists and few holistic practitioners were qualified to be certified.

This one-of-a-kind book was written by a certified holistic practitioner on the ancient art of ear candling.

The Institute of Certified Ear Candler's in Los Angeles, California, offers a nationwide distant learning course in less than forty hours that teaches the ear coning treatment that is just as beneficial today as it was centuries ago.

For the health-conscious individual who is fatigued with conventional methods and unnecessary ear surgery, and with drugs that have failed to excel the condition ear candling immediately provides; it is the best known treatment for the proper care of the outer ear canal. This ancient modality is a gentle, safe, and effective process that creates a calming mood that relieves stress and fatigue in adults, and settles anxiousness experienced by young children as early as thirty months of age. One ear cone per ear is ample, practical and safe for younger children.

Ear coning is a detoxification procedure that should be done annually since the ear has no natural process of elimination.

Penny Rich, CEC, CHt.
Certified Ear Coneologist

Chapter 1

In the Beginning

It was thousands of years ago in ancient cultures that ear coning, also known today as ear candling, was used to clean the outer ear canal where a powdery substance, candidacies (yeast), grows and thrives along the dark moist membrane walls inside the folds of skin consisting of the outer ear canal.

Turkish people may have been among the first to bring this procedure to the Middle East centuries after the Egyptian era. Beautiful young Thai girls cleaned ears in the local barbershops. The Indian culture gave its own specific touch to ear coning. It is said that men walked the streets with long instruments carried in their hat bands which they would whip out on the spur of the moment in the public square and clean ears for a penny-a-cone with amazing results.

Ear candling has been practiced for at least five centuries in the Far Eastern countries by many different cultures and is considered as necessary as personal hygiene required in maintaining healthy teeth and gums.

Ear candling is one of the oldest remedies for the treatment of *minor* ear maladies and falls into the category of holistic medicine. It is best performed by a qualified and trained technician known as an Ear Coneologist, a word coined by the Institute of Certified Ear Candler's at the turn of the century.

Treating the Outer Ear Canal

A normal substance known as candida is a fungus that consists of minute cells of bodily bacteria (microorganisms) that reproduces by budding and clumping together to form a gray to yellow, frothy, vicious growth. Over a period of time, they can cause disorders of the ear and other parts of both the female and male body. These abnormal fungi and debris create infectious toxicity that stems from liver and kidney bile found in the birth mother's embryonic fluids. It is most unfortunate that physicians do not clean the ears when we are born because the extremely delicate membrane could be irreversibly damaged.

These fragile mechanisms of balance and hearing are affected by these troublesome parasites, even though diseases are not generally as serious as those that develop inside the middle and inner ears. These are usually confined within the folds of skin, as well as in the cartilage found in the pinna (external ear).

Whenever we open our mouth to yawn, the ear canal opens and stretches, making it receptive to the invasion of foreign matter.

Adverse conditions that may be caused by these parasites can often lead to crippling diseases such as Bell's palsy, when the auditory nerve endings are damaged causing the facial muscles to become paralyzed. When candida has attached itself to the delicate auditory nerves that control them, these nerves extend from the brain through a small hole in the skull located just behind the ear where swelling begins. However, it is not yet known in the medical profession why these two facial nerves are thusly affected.

Medical students in Europe are required to learn this alternative method as a preventive measure.

Balance and Hearing

Since the brain is constantly monitoring movement of the head and body, balance is maintained when information to the brain is received; our eyes then coordinate the assimilated data that produces a state of equal balance, or equilibrium, a condition in which opposing forces balance equally to create a mental balance.

When candida and other infestations invade the outer ear, they begin to affect vision and hearing as well, causing balance to be impaired. Headaches, deafness, and even a reduction of the crystalline lens, located at the back of the head behind the eye socket, can be affected enough to cause blurred vision.

Ear candling can serve to relieve minor eye pressure and differentiate the perception of colors, making them appear to be sharper and brighter.

Who Needs Ear Candling?

Since 1996, the ear candling process has grown in popularity as people became more involved in holistic alternatives, as opposed to conventional medicine, in an effort to avoid doctors (who are indeed "practicing" physicians) who decide to make us candidates to participate in some kind of paid laboratory experiment, or to test a new drug on us which may result in a dozen or more disabling side effects.

Becoming more aware of the alternative health care methods could enable us to live longer, and to enjoy more productive lives.

So who needs ear candling? Let every human ear be thusly "pampered" for better health. We all need it—gardeners, ditch and grave diggers, garbage collectors, mail carriers, and construction workers. We all lure an abundance of dust and debris directly into the outer ear canal, just as those who work in less polluted environments such as the office, the supermarket, and the beauty salon attract pollutants en route to their workplace. While the left ear may also be more susceptible to collecting minute flying insects and dust when we drive with the window down. These too are literally expelled during the ear coning process along with excess ear wax.

Amazingly enough, Laurriet, my mother, had placed a cherry pit into her ear as a child, and it was not discovered for over fifty years. When her hearing became more impaired, she suffered with frequent earache until the tiny pit was removed by a medical physician. She had not realized her hearing was not as good as it could have been since such a long time had passed since she playfully pushed the seed into the outer ear where there is "no process of elimination."

It should not come as a surprise to learn that we are born with parasites inside our ears where mold and other normal infestation proliferate in darkness, subjecting the ears to fine particles that swoop inside grooves of skin in the outer ear, packing micro layers of matter—with as much as two teaspoons of toxic substance that is pushed deeper into the canal when you poke inside with Q-tips and other foreign objects. Inevitably, you will no longer be able to hear well.

There is yet only one safe and effective way that it may be removed—the holistic alternative, ear candling. It's a miraculous remedy that speaks well for itself.

Hearing Loss Problems

The primary purpose for the ear, for those who may still be wet behind them, is to modify and channel sound waves. These normal sound waves enter the ear canal causing the tympanic membrane (eardrum) to vibrate, setting in motion the tiny bones of the middle ear known as the hammer, anvil, and stirrup.

These tiny bones, the smallest in the entire body, magnify and transfer sounds to the structures of the inner ear known as the cochlea and auditory nerve. Inside the cochlea are tiny hairs that convert sounds to nerve impulses, which are transmitted to the brain via delicate nerve endings.

Today, with the pulsating blast of boom box's pounding to the loud music from car radios, these tiny hairs in the cochlea are rapidly breaking down due to exposure to constant rhythm of vibrating noises, and there is no way they will ever be revived.

Impaired hearing will result eventually, and the listener will not be capable of hearing the precious vibrations created by sound. The listener will require a hearing device, provided there is any level of hearing remaining since it is virtually impossible to reverse this kind of hearing loss.

Ear candling is a procedure that may instantly help relieve the symptoms of tiredness, as it lowers stress levels.

However, diet is a factor as well. Avoid too much salt, caffeine, alcohol, dairy products, and bread . . . but don't forget to treat yourself to a glass of chilled wine.

Smoking contributes to inflammation as it irritates mucous membranes that line the nose, so one should carefully consider what he puts up his nose.

When your pulse rate is fewer than 50 or more than 150 beats per minute, it is a wise man who immediately consults a medical doctor. Ear coning is not going to help you out of that one.

Serious Ear Infections and How to Avoid Them

When ear infections become serious enough to require the advice of a medical practitioner, the middle ear may be involved as well. First warning is pain and pressure inside the ear.

Middle ear infections usually start with a cold that may cause the Eustachian tube, a slender canal between the pharynx and the middle ear that leads to the throat), to close due to swelling. When this happens, air cannot reach the middle ear. Infections occur when bacteria or viruses develop and thrive in the existing fluid. Draining from the ear that is bloody or looks like pus may indicate a ruptured membrane or perforated eardrum

Ear coning treatments are not given to those with damaged eardrums without the consent of a medical physician—and *that* isn't going to happen.

Infection and inflammation can cause otitis-externa or "swimmer's ear" that develops after water, sand, and other foreign debris has entered the outer ear.

Swimmer's ear symptoms include pain, itching, and a feeling of fullness in the canal. It may become swollen and increase the agony of pain, discharge, and possible loss of hearing.

Constant probing with a cotton swab or some other object not intended to be put in the ear canal may cause inflammation. It is also best to avoid prolonged use of ear plugs, soap or shampoo buildup, and chronic skin conditions that could spread infections and contagious disease.

This information is given as a point of reference. Ear candling professionals neither diagnose, nor treat any medical problems.

Beginning Stages of Hearing Loss

Hearing loss is a common ailment, especially in adults over the age of fifty. By then, the buildup of toxic waste material has already begun its process of deterioration that leads to irreversible damage.

Certain medications including high doses of common household aspirin (eight to twelve tablets), along with changes that come with age, known as presbycusis that cause people to experience a loss of understanding of another person's conversation and still remain very sensitive to loud noises. They may also constantly hear ear ringing, hissing, or clicking sounds in the ear.

Hearing may also become impaired when something prevents sound from reaching the inner ear. This person is a perfect candidate for ear candling in the instance where packed ear wax can be easily removed to improve hearing.

Another cause for natural hearing loss is the presence of excess fluid in the middle or inner ear. When hearing loss is not treated, it contributes to depression, social isolation, and loss in self-dependence, especially in the elderly group. Some loss may be the result of decreased blood flow to the inner ear.

Frequently Asked Questions

"Is it true that all that 'stuff' that comes out of the candle comes out of my ears?" Definitely not!

Part of that material is residue from the burnt 100 percent muslin cloth from which the candle is made. You'll notice there are several different *colors and textures* in the pungent, frothy substance extracted from the ear canal. This mixture is a combination of candida, natural yeast-infested matter consisting of parasites, excess ear wax, fungi, debris, and decayed microorganisms from embryonic fluid that was never removed from your ears when the nurse cleaned your mouth and nose at birth.

As it increasingly becomes toxic, it may be the cause of lost brain cell activity, imbalance, unpleasant facial distortion, and bulging eyes.

Conventional methods are usually invasive and have been known to cause permanent damage to the ear's tympanic membrane (eardrum). Minor ear maladies that stem primarily from improper diet and swimming in polluted waters are best treated with ear candling that deals only with the outer ear canal. This is important to remember.

Where Does Candida Come From?

It's a natural phenomenon. We are born with it as it derives from the lifestyle and eating habits of our biological parents.

The toxins stem from a greenish fluid secreted by liver bile. This bile is passed on the moment we emerge from the womb. Once the membrane that surrounds the amniotic fluid pouch in which the infant floats breaks open, the risk of infection increases. The nurse immediately wipes mucus from the mouth and nose of the infant but never from the delicate ear canal itself where these parasitic fungi begin to develop and thrive in the dark moisture of specific areas of our bodies.

This dark, moist space becomes a breeding ground for disease that the unsuspecting parent has passed on to the child. Before a child reaches two or three years of age, fluid may have developed behind the eardrum that may seep into the outer ear canal in what appears to be a greenish fluid that can cause a child to be irritable.

How I Became a Certified Ear Coneologist

We all are aware that good things prosper by word of mouth. This is one service in which we are greatly impressed with the success ratio of the ear candling experience that lends itself to relaxation and relief from stress within the first fifteen minutes of a treatment.

I became involved in this particular holistic endeavor in 1996, when I found relief to a nagging headache at a dinner party where I was unexpectedly asked to follow my host, Pat, upstairs. She invited me to lie down on her bed so she could put a cone-shaped cylinder with a full ½ inch flame burning on one end into the opening of my external ear.

"I'm going to light this cone," Pat said, "and put it in your ear."

"You're going to do *what*?" I quickly responded.

"It'll take away your headache right away . . . lie on your side," she continued. "and let your other ear be toward the ceiling. You're going to love it."

My mother and twin sister looked on with bated breath as I became her guinea pig. I'd hardly had time in my life to travel to foreign countries to ever see such a thing being done but I didn't give it a second thought. Within minutes of the brief session, my headache was gone, and I wouldn't think about it again for a couple of weeks.

While going through another "burnt-out" phase of my wallpaper hanging business, which I'd done on several occasions only to dig in deeper, the thought occurred to me that I might enjoy sharing the unusual ear cleaning treatment with others and decided to give it some serious consideration. I had no doubt it wasn't a darn good idea because I was impressed with the results after only a few minutes of the treatment. Why else would I tackle it on a larger scale if I didn't think it would work?

A few days later, while hanging paper in three bathrooms in the Pacific Palisades, I told my client, Linda, a doctor's wife, that I was ready to retire and that no one was giving me a retirement party or a gold watch after twenty-five years In the business at that time. That evening when I finished the job, we toasted its completion with a glass of champagne.

Arriving home quite late, I flopped down on the sofa, very tired and exhausted. I had to finish the job because I didn't want to drive out there again the next day. Four days was enough! I was almost ready to retire . . . again.

I knew if I sat there any longer, I'd soon be fast asleep. Suddenly, that sweet voice of intuition inside my head told me to get up and go to bed or I'd still be sitting there and very cold by the early hours of dawn.

Painfully I struggled to get up, but I couldn't. Every muscle in my body had shut down. I was so tired, I wanted to cry. This wasn't an unfamiliar situation for me. I worked very hard all the time because I'm a perfectionist, and my work represented that of a skilled master of her trade.

Then clearly, the idea occurred to me that I needed to think about doing something else as a vocation . . . but what? It was then that a light came on in my head. Ear coning! Yes! I said to myself. "I'll find out what I need the first thing in the morning and I'll launch an ear coning business."

The moment ear coning became an option, I immediately rose from the corner of the sofa without one single sign of a muscle spasm or pain, showered, and went to bed . . . with a smile on my face.

I woke earlier than usual and began to compile all the information I could find on ear coning, but there was very little positive information available on the internet.

I put together what items I could remember from the short session my friend, Pat, offered—scissors, cotton balls, aluminum bowl for water, a lighter, virgin olive oil, a large candle, a clear glass jar for the waste material, a few hand towels, and a large canvas bag to hold everything in.

All I needed now were the candles, as Pat made excuses on a daily basis to avoid giving me her source until she finally gave me the name of the man who made them for her.

It was during that long wait that I had a chance to do some dedicated research on ear candling combining the medical aspects of the human ear with holistic facts.

After months of actual treatments that followed, I knew about as much as I could from doing the ears of several friends and family members and was ready to take on my first real client. I made an appointment with a friend who was actually the first person who informed me that her color perception had vastly improved when she noticed that the trees outside her living window appeared to be brighter and sharper. It would be the first of many annual treatments for her and her elderly mother over the years that followed.

Oh, you should have seen me! I wore all white; blouse, pants, shoes, socks and a smock with my "new" company name, Institute of Certified Ear Candler's, embroidered on the back. The hand-printed name, "Penny" was written across the breast pocket. I wore a cute "Big Apple" similar to the one known as a "newspaper boy's" cap that was so popular in the 1940s. I carried my tools in a small carry-on with wheels. *That* was over twenty-two years ago. The rest is history.

I'll never forget how proud of myself I was, and probably feeling a new surge of creative energy I hadn't felt in years!

Ten years later, I founded the only state registered program to teach ear coning through a nationwide home study course which was running concurrently with my wallpaper installation business until I retired in 2007.

Now the question was, how was I going to promote this bizarre modality that seemed to heal some of the most common maladies—in the real world? It had been months of actual experience that turned out to be the best teacher promoted by word-of-mouth.

As I stared at the neat coning kit I'd put together, it dawned upon me that I needed to find a way to get the word out. At the time, it was still a very controversial treatment. How would I convince folks to let me put a burning candle into their ears?

Determining a marketing strategy was the next step. The word "media" popped out, and I picked up the telephone and contacted KCAL-9 News, a local television station. Almost as if I was being guided along, I stopped thinking and placed a call an anonymous caller who had just witnessed the most bizarre-looking treatment (across the street) that I'd ever seen! I panted with excitement and believability as I described to the (former) reporter, Gay Yee, what appeared to be something she had never seen or heard of before either. Much to my surprise, she was very interested in holistic alternatives. The call had peeked her interest and within minutes, she was asking questions about how she could get in touch with the "lady across the street"—me.

Her name is Penny . . . Penny Rich . . . p-e-n-n-y-r-i-c-h, I spelled slowly and then gradually put my own phone number together as if trying to remember it as she jotted down the vital information.

As soon as she verified my information, I quickly excused myself, telling her that I was going back across the street because "people were starting to line up over there."

At nine o'clock the next morning, the phone rang. It was Ms Yee. "Good morning. Did someone there call the Channel 9 newsroom?" she asked.

"No," I lied politely. "May I help you?"

"Well, is there someone there who knows about the treatment that puts fire in the ear?" she continued, sounding a bit disappointed.

"Yes," I replied with more interest. "I'm Penny Rich. The treatment is called ear coning."

While I was explaining the ancient remedy, she was taking notes after which she asked if they could do a news segment on me,—and scheduled an interview the following Tuesday for the ten o'clock news.

I was so busy trying to remain composed that I thought she said, "Thursday."

Tuesday morning the crew arrived at a neighborhood beauty salon on La Brea near 8th Street, the location I'd given for the shoot. Ms. Yee wasn't too happy that I was not there yet. She called and I told her I was on my way. I'd just gotten out of bed a half hour earlier, but I was only five minutes away.

When I arrived, the camera crew was all set up and waiting for me. The owner's daughter sat in a barber's chair as I presented the demonstration on ear candling.

I'll always remember how dramatic the reporter was. At the end of the segment, she tagged it with the words, "It seems to me . . . that Penny Rich . . . is playing . . . with fire!"

On Channel 9 throughout the following day, still shots aired that showed me holding a candle in the ear of my client with a reminder to tune in to the ten o'clock news to find out more about the very "controversial" treatment known as ear coning. It finally aired at 10:20 p.m. How exciting was *that*?

I called the next morning to get some feedback on the response they had received. When I asked if she would add another phone number (instead of a message number I'd given to Ms Yee), she said, "Is *this* Penny Rich?"

"Yes," I replied.

"Let me tell 'ya! We took so many calls after your story aired last night that we're going to repeat it on the twelve o'clock noon news today," she said excitedly.

However, by this time, they were no longer calling the ancient remedy "controversial." It was an instant hit! It had indeed "grown by popular demand" . . . overnight.

That so-called anonymous phone call set into motion the beginning of a very successful new venture.

My moment of *creative advertising* and *invaluable publicity* had brought the treatment into full focus.

A Leap of Faith

I was suddenly swamped with appointments as I made my living room, a temporary office with folks coming and going within twenty minutes of each other with just enough time between sessions to refreshen up the area.

With such an excellent response, I was inspired to to inquire about a booth at the upcoming Black Business Conference for a two-day weekend show at the Los Angeles Convention Center downtown.

Since that was the weekend of the conference, I was informed that all the booths were sold out, however, a well-known vendor had canceled and had forfeited their five-hundred dollar deposit. It was a choice corner 10x10 booth with two long tables and two chairs for eleven-hundred dollars from which she deducted the previous deposit and offered it to me for six hundred dollars. All I had to do was bring her an additional two-hundred dollars and have the balance of four-hundred the next morning before the show . . . . with a warning: I would not be able to get my deposit back if I didn't pay it.

"No problem," I replied . . . even though I didn't have that kind of money lying around, but, that didn't stop me. This was a tremendous opportunity to present the most interesting and unique treatment that had been exposed to the media.

I wrote a check for the balance and just knew that by Monday, I would have enough in my account to clear it. (In those days, the bank system shut down for the week-end and there was no way to verify funds). She trusted me and I had every intention to honor my commitment. This was truly "a leap of faith".

People were standing three-deep around my booth, looking over each other's shoulders trying to see the lady putting fire into the ears of the curious "guinea pigs" who were brave enough to let me treat them as I extracted a substance that looked like powdered mustard from their ears.

A Change of Plan

Just before September 11, 2001, I had scheduled an ear coning health seminar at a popular health food store in Greensboro, North Carolina, through a friend (Josie) whom I'd met when she was visiting in California on business but then came that unforgettable morning I'd been awakened by the story of the terrorist attack on the World Trade Center in the heart of New York City. It was like an unbelievably horrific nightmare brought to life. I had totally forgotten the ear coning presentation in Greensboro. I was not about to get on a plane to go anywhere!

The phone rang a few days later. It was one of the five ladies interested in learning the art of the ancient ear coning remedy. She was very disappointed at my not showing up. It was that very moment I suggested she take my "home study course" for two-hundred-fifty dollars for which she would receive our enrollment packet. Well, at the time, I didn't have a home study course; but by midnight that evening, I did! I immediately revised the book I'd written on ear candling, *Pamper Your Ears with Fire!*, adding the words *The Ear Candler's Manual* that has been on sale at the Bodhi Tree Book Store in West Hollywood since 1989. It is still the only book available with comprehensive information about the treatment and everything I could find on the outer ear canal. It had suddenly been transformed into a textbook.

Seven years later, the state of California would increase our forty-hour study and certification requirement into a twelve-hundred-fifty dollar course requiring it to be a full-time school operation for California-based students that was supposed to be completed in as little as six months, but since there wasn't enough data to substantiate such a long-term program, we went *nationwide* to provide a distant learning program where students from around the world have enrolled in and graduated as certified ear coneologists. A few years later, I was invited to travel to South Korea where I was given an opportunity to present the treatment to several Buddhist priests (and their wives) in my room at the fabulous five-star hotel, the Lotte, in Seoul. They watched with much interest, after which I was given the distinction of bringing ear coning to South Korea where (to the best of my knowledge) it is still being used.

By the time I arrived home, there was a large order for ear candles to be sent to Seoul to the priest, a bachelor, who was always on the tour bus in the seat next to mine. They only needed *one cone* as a sample, and my supply source became instantly nullified.

Over the past years, we have certified one hundred and fifty-two students from Seattle to Canada, from Nevada to Hawaii, and now, Belmont, Australia through our California based website.

Every human being in the world is meant to enjoy good hearing and balance when the ear is properly maintained with a cleaning that provides the ultimate solution for the entire family from two and a half years old to the elderly population for which there seems to be a strong connection to Alzheimer's disease and loss of memory with the slow deterioration of brain cell activity caused by the toxicity of the proliferation of yeast and debris found just inside the ear.

Ear candling is this century's oldest procedure that is just as beneficial today as it was during the Egyptian era with only one difference: it has become a common household word in the twenty-first century.

What Did the Doctor Say?

Shortly after the airing of our television news segment, the reporter paid a visit to a Beverly Hills physician, Dr. Robert Nemeroff, ENT, who was asked what he personally thought about ear candling, to which he replied, (quote) "Ear wax does serve as a protective role in fighting off infections. One, because of its pH factor, and it has antibacterial and antifungal components, and clearly, if it was a very effective treatment that showed a lot of promise, we'd still be using it today!"

Well, Doctor, how can the pH factor be balanced if the ear is packed with candida and debris that causes major problems in folks of all ages, especially in youngsters who constantly suffer with earache and share the same cold germs with classmates at school?

When I was asked what I would say to other medical practitioners who would oppose the ear coning concept, I did not hesitate to reply, "Doctor, lend me your ears."

When I called the ENT's office the following day, my offer to clean his ears was, of course, rejected.

How Does the Ear Cone Work?

This ancient remedy works with the use of a handmade, cylinder-shaped, thirteen-inch cone made from unbleached 100 percent muslin cloth that has been saturated in 100 percent beeswax, shaped on a stick and hung up to dry.

Gently placed just inside the outer (external) ear canal, coning allows the larger end of the cylinder to burn safely as it extracts a toxic, odiferous, powdery substance that has most likely existed since you left the comfort of your mother's womb.

Ear candling provides excellent results in the improvement, care, enhancement, and maintenance of the canal. It is a safe, painless, and effective holistic alternative to conventional medicine. Although it is still being frowned upon by the medical profession due to the controversy surrounding its widespread use, several medical physicians have adobted its use in their offices over the past few years as an *effective preventative measure*. This is a sure sign that there are some who have the best interest of their patient's (pocket-books) at heart. Seemingly, some unnecessary surgical procedures are costing the government a tremendous amount of money.

A form of acupressure does the work as a steady flow of smoke produces a swirling vapor bath that gently expels matter into the cone and then it is tapped out in two fifteen—minute intervals per cone, thus, the two-hour relaxing and most effectively beneficial treatment. Anyone offering a one-cone-per-ear treatment is wasting your time as the toxic substance lies just inside the external ear causing itching along with the temptation to insert any conveniently available foreign object into the outer ear canal for fast relief that can be avoided.Since bodily functions respond to pressure points surrounding the external ear, smoke creates a gentle vacuum that extracts candida infestation and other debris. This gentle osmosis effect seems to equalize ear pressure, steady balance, and improve hearing loss as the natural cone slowly burns down to a safe distance away from the external ear in two segment cuts of the (fire-line) safety marked on the Best Quality Ear Cone.

When candling, we look for the lighter textures and coloring to be the most decayed matter. The lighter the substance, the more toxic it tends to produce because it's been there the longest, while the darker lighter gold colored matter may consist of wax flakes, flying insects, fungus, or mold that may also contain high levels of toxic waste.

As this residue becomes crystallized, it becomes extremely odiferous and can make a room smell like a morgue if the jar is left uncovered for several hours. This concoction should be discarded *immediately* since it is dangerously unhealthy to inhale the vapors that escape.

What emerges from this frothy substance of candida and other microorganisms is the total history of the way you live—determined by your environment, diet, medications, drugs, and alcohol consumption.

What it creates is the result of years of decaying infestation that has literally developed into human toxic waste that causes a myriad of ear, nose and throat maladies, colds, and unnecessary illness.

Medical vs. Holistic:

How Medical Physicians Feel about Ear Coning

With any problem related to the outer ear canal, the middle or inner ear, it is always best to consult a medical doctor since what we may determine to be a "minor' problem is predicated on the simplicity of the feeling that is usually annoying or aggravating.

Symptoms such as ear pain, fever, difficulty in chewing, headache, pressure in the ear, stuffy nose, persistent cough, hearing loss, dizziness or light-headedness, nose bleeding and Vertigo, is a strong indication that a medical physical should be contacted as this may indicate more serious problems than a malady of the outer ear showing signs of minor physical discomfort.

Vertigo, Dizziness, and Balance Disorders

These are two symptoms that describe two different conditions related to the outer ear.

Vertigo is a sensation that makes you feel like the room is spinning around when your eyes are closed and when there is no actual movement of the body.

Vertigo may also be caused by labyrinthitis, an inflammation or infection in the part of the inner ear that controls balance usually caused by a viral infection that usually follows the flu or a lingering cold with other underlying problems such as multiple sclerosis, stroke, and, in some rare cases, brain tumor.

Dizziness or light-headedness is a sensation that makes you feel faint like you're ready to pass out. Even though you may feel off balanced, there is no sensation of movement. It is a feeling slightly similar to how you may feel after an ear coning treatment corrected by drinking a glass of water immediately thereafter to balance the median. Water or juice replenishes the feeling of emptiness or lightness in the head.

Other causes of light-headedness may include alcohol, drugs, hyperventilation, stress, anxiety, fatigue, and blood loss. It could also be a momentary drop in blood pressure and reduced blood flow to the head when rising or getting up from a seated or lying position too quickly.

This sensation is called orthostatic hypotension and may also be caused by dehydration, medication, certain prescribed blood pressure, and heart medications.

Recurrent spells of serious light-headedness and dizziness can lead to fainting spells known as cardiac syncope. Unexplained fainting spells need to be evaluated by a medical physician or specialist immediately.

More serious vertigo problems often related to inner ear problems are not uncommon with cold or flu and allergies symptoms.

Ear candling is not a medical remedy, I'll repeat. It is holistic and does not require topical medications and drugs. The medical profession does not openly or fully recognize ear candling as an effective method of cleaning the ear canal. They seem to prefer to make incisions into the eardrum (myringotomy procedure) in order to drain fluids from behind the tympanic membrane by inserting a tiny ventilating tube.

However, during the healing process, candida is still building up. When the tube falls out, it is usually replaced. Infections are treated with antibiotics. When this method of perforation of the eardrum is unsuccessful, infection may invade the bone around the mastoid cells. The mastoid is the projection of bone behind the ear where the tiniest bones in the entire body are. When this occurs, acute mastoiditis may cause swelling behind the ear, high fever, and other signs of a major problem. This particular operation is common practice and can be costly.

Again, we are not medical practitioners. Do not consider this to be medical advise under any circumstance.

The most common balance disorder is Meniere's disease which is believed to be caused by a buildup of fluid in the inner ear with symptoms that include attacks of unsteadiness, tinnitus, hearing loss in one ear, and may sometimes cause nausea and vomiting, which represents a serious problem for medical diagnoses, especially when standing or walking seems impossible.

Drugs That Can Damage the Ear

With continued research, we have also learned that many drugs and antibiotics prescribed by medical physicians can cause damage to the structures and functions of the ear. Those considered more toxic seem to attack the hair cells of the cochlea and cause the inability to discriminate high tones are as follows: neomycin, kanamycin, dihydrostreptomycin, and vancomycin. Medications that end with the word "mycin" are antibiotics to support hearing loss in degrees of their severity.

These damaging drugs buildup in the bloodstream where there is a decrease in healthy kidney functions, allowing the process of irreversible damage to accelerate. When there is a problem of vertigo, a doctor may prescribe one or more drugs that will affect balance before it affects hearing.

Streptomycin and gentomycin can both cause loss of coordination by destroying the hair cells of the balance organ. Once vertigo has stopped, a sense of equilibrium occurs. However, if the use of drugs continues, nerve deafness may result as the auditory labyrinth becomes involved.

Incidentally, without a natural process of elimination, all meds remain in the delicate mechanisms of the ear for an undetermined amount of time as an unknown factor to be adjusted in time.

It is vital that we utilize the past to ease the maladies of our future. Others in the medical field will hopefully someday realize the true value and importance of maintaining good health through tried practices that are less costly, less invasive, and yet substantially more effective and beneficial as found in holistic alternatives.

Fortunately, our western culture has expanded its knowledge of holistic treatment to include the lost art of ear candling, thanks to devoted lawmakers who implemented the rules and regulations that brought political change that we might precede with the healing of mankind.

Ear Coning and How it Benefits Cocaine and Other Substance Users

People who are subject to drug abuse of any kind, who have a desire to rid themselves of illegal substance, have found ear candling the most successful in matching that goal by eliminating the sensory perception of substances remaining on the roof of the mouth as a constant reminder of its taste and smell. This is the same area in which toxins and other "reminders" coat the tongue.

However, when the taste is removed from the lymphatic, the sensory system, and the tongue has been cleaned, such cravings are greatly diminished.

Another power tool for making subconscious changes is hypnosis. Oriental herbs are additional remedies that encourage long-term abstinence.

The Pioneer Who Met the Challenge–Diane E. Watson, PHd

My most respected peer and the pioneer to whom we, as holistic practitioners, will forever be grateful is the former congresswoman, Diane E. Watson, who fought for our right to choose alternatives to conventional medicine.

As an advocate for holistic health rights and benefits, she was instrumental in helping those of us who had become somewhat disenchanted with conventional methods of simple health care and maintenance to obtain national recognition and support in matters relating to holistic endeavors starting with California residents.

With insight, concern, and a passionate love for humanity, Dr. Watson blazed a trail for those who would prefer avenues of self-healing of the mind and body with freedom of choice in making alternative health care decisions.

The Ear and Its Vital Points

The human ear represents every vital point in the human body. In stimulating these potent focal points in the outer ear canal with warmth created by a flame on the large end of the ear cone, we trigger the release of endorphins that provide relaxation and release daily stress factors.

Some benefits produced by acupressure are the management of stress and a heightened mental clarity that seems to deepen spiritual awareness.

Many of our clients have extraordinary clairvoyant abilities that are even more enhanced as continued treatments appear to open their *charka* with the removal of toxicity produced by the growth and proliferation of yeast infestation.

Vision is improved as the weight of the toxic substance is lifted from the crystalline lens located in the back of the head behind the eye socket and taste buds are better receptive to define the flavors of food.

Chapter II

Purpose of ICEC

Institute of Certified Ear Candler's

The primary reason for establishing the Institute of Certified Ear Candler's in 2000 was to reach out to those all around the world who were interested in the continuation of this effective and beneficial procedure.

The ICEC distant learning course is intended to train and certify professional, qualified holistic practitioners in the area of ear cleaning, ear care, and maintenance as ear coneologists, to teach the basic elements of the outer ear, specializing in comprehensive knowledge regarding proper procedures and health-related precautions. By the turn of the twenty-first century, over 1,500 hours had spanned a twenty-two-year period. Being dedicated to the practical use of alternatives along with the loving concern for the health of others, ICEC has certified between seven and eight hundred students since 1995.

With proper instructions, you are assured that you will experience positive results. With a success ratio of 98.8 percent, verified by testimonials and case histories, it is no surprise that actual experience in the field had indeed been the best teacher in a practical remedy that dates back many centuries.

Perhaps a few of those who had been more than curious, with a prior interest in the benefits of ear coning, were discouraged and misled by medical practitioners who knew absolutely zero about its use and proven benefits.

Ear candling is a holistic remedy for minor ear maladies in children as early as two and half years old. The older we get, the more toxicity has built up, making us perfect candidates for outer ear canal problems such as Bell's palsy and beginning phases (through research) of dementia and Alzheimer's disease.

Each of the six cones used, three per ear, are burned down approximately three inches to four inches from the ear, which is a pretty safe distance as not to feel any warmth from the burning end of the candle.

Benefits include the improvement of:

Hearing loss, Balance disorders and helps to decrease minor incidents of sinus congestion, ear ringing, allergies and cold symptoms, vertigo, swimmer's ear, dizziness, Bell's palsy, migraine headache and color perception making things appear to be sharper and brighter.

- While is also improves areas of the sinus and nasal cavity
- Affords increased feelings of vitality
- Emotional release of toxins as they leave the body
- Brighter tones in hearing quality
- Notable distinction of mental clarity
- Equilibrium/Relief of ear pressure

The Ear Candling Procedure

It has been revealed that ear coning was in use during the Egyptian era. As to exactly how this "vacuum cleaner" for the ears works remains a mystery. How well it works is yet quite amazing!

Ear coning is just as effective now as it was when newspaper was coiled up tightly and placed into the outer ear canal. As it burnt, a smoke-vapor bath pulled substances out and cleared the passage to improve hearing and balance disorders, producing a feeling of cleanliness as it released toxins debris.

Today, a handmade cone (or cylinder) has replaced quick burning newspaper with a safe, comfortable, and natural tool that works to improve several related symptoms pertaining to the eyes, nose, and throat.

Apparently, there is nothing new under the sun, especially in areas of holistic medicine.

Herbs have been in use since the beginning of time, and with the increased use of oriental medicine and other natural alternatives and remedies, a new light shines on the subject of self-preservation that may put needless surgery and drugs in the dark.

The herb Echinacea is often used in some candles that may cause it to slowly relieve the density of the yeast that has proliferated. ICEC recommends the *Best Quality* Ear Cone as it is all-natural and works well for very sensitive sinus congestion symptoms.

It is preferred that you are relaxed and comfortable in a peaceful, quiet, and well-ventilated environment, while a professional ear coneologist provides the service for you.

What to Look Forward To

In a reclining position while the subject is lying preferably on a portable (light-weight) massage table, the opposite ear is on a firm pillow, the ear is ready to receive the twelve-inch to thirteen-inch ear candle as it can only work properly when the ear is horizontal so that the smoke can circulate through the cylinder. The cone must be held in an (almost) upright (eleven o'clock) position extended above the ear.

The larger end of the cone is aflame in order to produce smoke that fills the cone in gentle circulating rolls of smoke patterns that are slightly visible through the thin, cloth-based ear cone, guided directed slightly into the opening of the ear canal toward the tympanic membrane from which it returns and pulls with it, a substance that appears to be similar to powdered mustard with bits and pieces of various kinds of waste material, including excess ear wax and yeast. This in itself is a cultural shock if you've never seen it before.

With the smaller end of the cone placed inside the external ear and gently held by your technician, the smoke travels downward, entering the canal in a swirling motion.

This treatment does not work if the individual being treated is sitting in a chair. It is scientifically impossible for the smoke to travel inward and work directly through the canal from that position. Remember, the cone is never forced inside the ear as only the orifice needs be closed to capture the vapor bath of the gentle smoke. There is absolutely no pain involved during the treatment.

A small pillow may be placed between the knees for additional comfort of the client.

During the process of reversed osmosis, you will hear a muted sound similar to a crackling fireplace on a cold night or the sound of a seashell nestled snuggly against your ear.

After approximately seven and a half minutes, the burning end is doused (head down) into the water to extinguish the flame. Always hold the candle down so as not to let water go inside the cone; it is not necessary to dip the entire blackened end of the candle into the aluminum bowl. The flame will extinguish immediately upon contact with the water.

Gently tap the candle over the water with your skewer tool until a slender roll of beeswax falls into the bowl. Cut off the burnt end then tap the powdery substance into your glass jar, tap gently along the length of the candle until it is empty. Relight the candle, and proceed with the same process.

You will have two cuts per candle prior to tapping the toxic matter into the glass jar. Proceed with two more candles; this process takes approximately one hour per ear.

When finished, clean exterior ear with alcohol squeezed from the cotton swab. Be sure ear-ring holes have been sanitized as well.

Then the person receiving the treatment is asked to gently clean inside his own ear with a Q-tip. Yes, a Q-tip, but not longer than five or six seconds. When the Q-tip appears to be clean, the canal usually is. Any time longer than a few seconds may cause the ear to feel irritated. Just go in and gently twirl the Q-tip around for a few seconds and then take it out. Not more than two or three Q-tips should be necessary. Too much probing into "virgin" ears will make them feel sensitive and uncomfortable.

In appearance, the candida (yeast) that comes from the ear is similar to crumbled, overcooked, hardboiled egg, or ground mustard, that normally builds up to trap infectious matter throughout your life. Remember, the ear is the only organ in the human body that does not have a process of elimination.

From birth and long before the age of puberty, the ear reacts to common ailments that affect every part of the body, especially the respiratory system.

The outer ear directly affects the nasal and sinus cavities or air space located behind the nose. This dedicated space is the main corridor to the respiratory system. When chronic infections spread to the middle ear, they may become acute due to excessive moisture or pressure as the virus dumps into the mastoid process located at the base of the external earlobe.

During cold or windy weather, it is suggested that a cotton ball be temporarily placed inside the ear for further comfort after a treatment. The ear canal should remain dry for at least twelve hours before washing hair or taking a shower.

The use of three cones per ear is highly recommended in order to take advantage of the pulling up and out of the waste material that clogs the outer ear canal as soft and frothy residue.

The treatment requires approximately two relaxing and pleasant hours to complete depending on the density of the contents that is being extracted and deposited into a dedicated small jar. However, when the ear cones have been kept in the freezer compartment of your refrigerator prior to use, the entire procedure is cut by about fifteen minutes. Perhaps it has something to do with the compression of the cotton fibers that the cone is made of.

When smoke appears to be coming from the burning end of the cone, it may be temporarily congested. Remove cone, push skewer through, and gently replace cone into canal and continue making adjustments that prevent extra smoke from escaping. When smoke escapes, the cone itself is merely burning away. Avoid drafts of wind flaming the candle. This will cause the candle to burn too rapidly and not treat effectively.

At the completion of the treatment, while the subject is still draped about the shoulders and head with a cloth to protect from an occasional drip of candle wax, she may be asked to sit up for a few seconds to make sure the ears feel open and refreshed. If there appears to be any mild pressure or discomfort, an extra ear cone would be appreciated—without extra charge. Simply repeat the clearing process again.

There is always some beneficial and noticeable feeling to be experienced after the treatment.

Again, *Best Quality Ear Cones* made especially for ICEC are engineered to withdraw toxic matter through a vacuuming process that filters out debris, parasites, fungi, microorganisms, and yeast. The darker bits and pieces may be considered ear cone residue from the cone itself, while the lighter difference in coloration is from the human ear as it appears to be the oldest substance being eliminated.

The most effective result of the ear candling experience comes from the circulation of smoke created by the ear cone; therefore, using only one cone per ear is neither effective nor beneficial.

The Human Ear's Mastoid Process

The mastoid is formed like a soft, fallen breast. The mastoid process found behind the nipple-shaped portion of the temporal bone extends downward and forward behind the external auditory meatus. The air spaces inside the mastoid process are called cells. Inflammation of these air cells is called mastoiditis.

Favorable Benefits of Ear Coning

Removal of the toxic substance alleviates disorders that may even cause loss of memory that we attribute to brain cell deterioration due to active toxins and the proliferation of odiferous yeast.

Removal helps renew youthfulness and feelings of vitality while it nurtures the mind and sensory perception.

The ear candling experience helps maintain balance, coordination, and motor skills; soothes the nerves; and decreases toxicity throughout the body. Once levels of toxicity are removed from the head, the body may feel healthier.

The Ear Has No Natural Process of Elimination

The sole avenue of elimination for the ear is not through the bowels, urinary tract, or glands. There is none. As much as 70 percent of body toxins exit through the surface of the skin, as during perspiration, and even more so through the feet during a foot and body detoxification procedure.

The lymphatic system dumps into the Eustachian or auditory tube that leads to the cavity behind the nose and permits equalization of air pressure on the outside. Sometimes, this tube becomes blocked due to a common cold. As it becomes clear the sudden burst of equalization of pressure feels like the ears have popped.

The ear candling cleansing process pulls debris out of these tubes, including the sinus and tear duct cavities. The outer ear also has a layer of skin that has no way to process elimination. The debris, fungi, and parasites find their home there, and at some point eventually may cause major problems that could have been prevented through holistic measures.

During the process, we look for the lighter gray matter to be the most toxic. As this residue becomes crystallized, it becomes a whiter-gray and extremely odiferous when removed and should be immediately discarded for the sake of good health.

When clients want to preserve it to show and tell, it is not recommended as it is unsafe to inhale these invisible fumes. Discard in a plastic or paper sack outside in a trash receptacle away from snooping animals.

A Special Kodak Moment

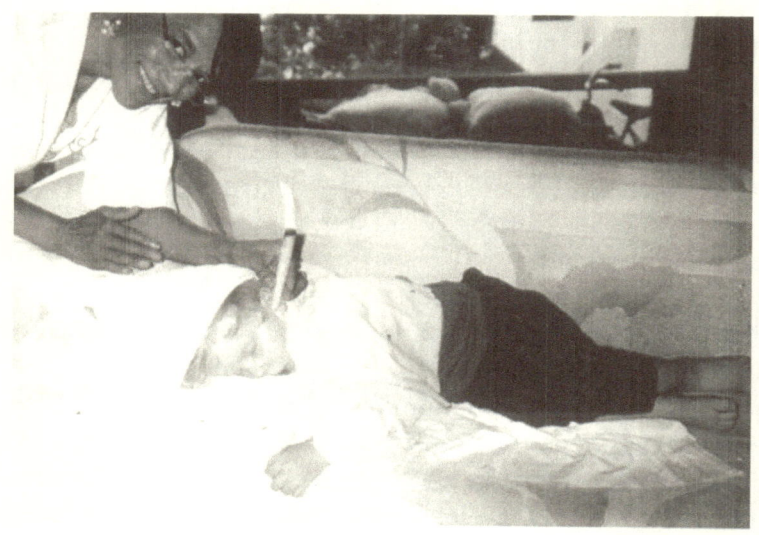

Child lying on sofa having an ear coning treatment as he sleeps

This baby's ears were treated when he was only two and a half years old. After watching the flame on the far end of the cone as his mother was being treated, you can imagine the fuss he made when it was his turn. She diverted his attention with his favorite toy, and the pleasant and relaxing sound in his ears lured him to sleep.

The child's presenting problem was a mild ear infection. Fluids had accumulated behind his eardrum, preventing the tympanic membrane from moving normally. His mother noticed green mucus on his pillow and that he had been unusually grumpy for several days.

Medical professionals warn us not to put any object into the ear that might perforate the eardrum. However, they feel qualified to remove this fluid by a procedure known as a "myringotomy" in which a tiny incision is made in the eardrum to promote drainage and the equalization of ear pressure. After a period of antibiotics, the incision is closed. Ear candling provides a safe, immediate solution without surgery.

The Cover-Up

Early in my ear candling procedure, I had failed to cover up my hair, my nose, and my mouth. Invisible debris from the smoke vapor is airborne, and those areas should be protected from them reentering the body through the nose and throat.

I was invited to have my hair follicles read by Dr. Kim at his holistic facility in Los Angeles. Yes, "read." It's another way to determine how healthy you are.

The doctor informed me that I had traces of diabetes and lupus in my chart.

For a few scary moments of bewilderment, I did not recall the previous day that I had treated a very unhealthy woman and her unhealthy teenage son in their home, not realizing the dangers I had exposed myself to. I had not covered my hair, nor was I wearing a filtering mask during either session. I suddenly felt sick over the mere idea. I was totally oblivious to any such contamination as traits of their symptoms had attached to my hair follicles.

Needless to say, I spent the next two hours at the hair salon.

The following day, Dr. Kim retested my hair and sure enough, my health had drastically improved!

Anyone in the same room should also be protected from airborne particles. Babies and smaller children should not be present at all.

Chapter III

Facts About Ear Wax

During the research stages of the Institute of Certified Ear Candler's, we discovered that over one million years ago, this planetary system was registered as an "inhibited world" when a mutation within the stock of the progressing primate suddenly produced two primitive human beings who were known as the ancestors of mankind. Fact or theory? In any event, ears have been around since the beginning of time. Although our bodies have become perfected in human concept, we haven't changed much in form for countless years.

In this major passage of time, this innovative age of lucrative business has buried the use of basic ancient remedies that were used generations ago. When our ancestors had problems with their ears, it was most likely the old, known, and proven cleansing methods of the Egyptian era with the use of fire that proved to be the most practical since most of them are still being used today.

Further research showed the ear canal as consisting of four thousand pores in each ear that produces, through certain glands, enough ear wax to provide the correct pH factor for an entire lifetime. Ear wax is produced twenty-four hours a day, seven days a week, three hundred sixty-five days a year. It is not likely that we will ever run short of it. The human body will help produce the exact amount needed and required to sustain healthy ears.

Ear Wax (Cerumen) Blockage

The medical term for ear wax is *cerumen*, which plays a vital part in protecting the ear canal. However, since ear wax replenishes itself within hours of removal of the old hardened wax chips that no longer serve a useful purpose, the amount may vary from one person to another. When blockage occurs, the ear feels clogged. Thus, mild congestion can result with partial loss of hearing, ear ringing sounds, and annoying ear pressure pain during flights that can also cause unnecessary pressure that can be very painful.

According to the American Medical Association, "the best self-help is prevention."

Water-Related Infections

While swimming, generalized infections can affect the entire skin lining of the outer ear canal. Excess moisture and polluted water, is a direct contact with parasites that live in bodies of water and thrive in the yeast fungi in the human ear.

Preventive measure: One should always avoid scratching inside the ear or probing with foreign objects for relief of itching. The itch simply indicates a need to clean the outer ear canal, possibly utilizing the safest and proven to be the most effective, beneficial alternative in holistic medicine.

Ear coning: This ancient remedy provides healthier hearing and balance all year around. Treatment may be scheduled once or twice a year at your convenience unless an urgency occurs.

Ear candling tends to place moderation and relief of infection and disease stemming from the inability to properly remove "excess baggage" from the outer ear canal.

When antibiotics are unsuccessful, surgery may be recommended by a medical practitioner who is opposed to holistic medicine and unaware of the miraculous benefits provided by the incredible ear coning experience.

Most often, the cause of the problem can be resolved with less expense and considerably less irreversible damage to the ear.

It has been proven throughout the holistic community that the best and most practical way to treat common ear infections in children, as well as adults of all ages, has been around longer than any of us can recall.

Medicine may relieve discomfort and mucus discharge for a short period, but when it dries, it can further clog the canal and present even more serious side effects.

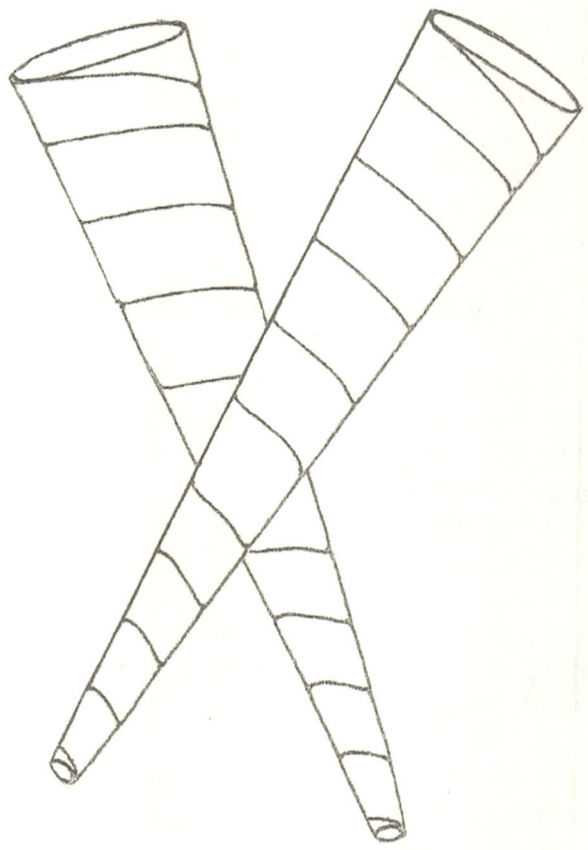

The Ear Cone

The ear cone used at ICEC is handmade
from 100 percent muslin, an unbleached cotton
material saturated in 100 percent beeswax. This
original, all-natural best quality ear cone
has no herbal enhancements or incense
to cause an allergenic reaction.
(*Not actural size*)

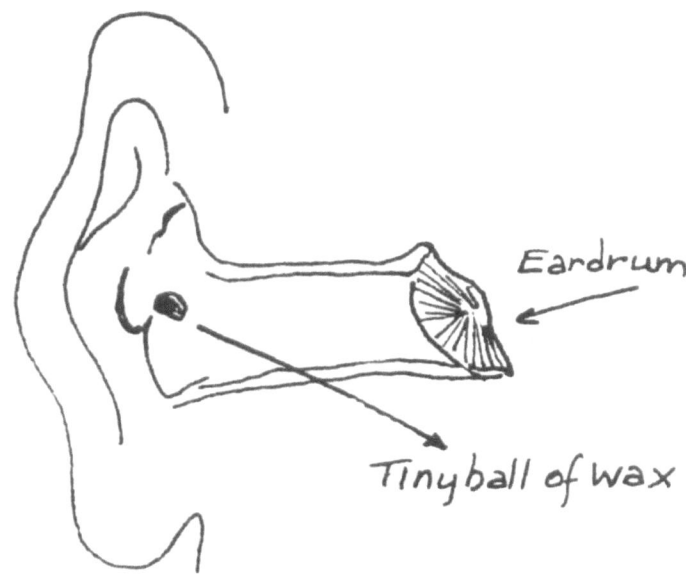

Eardrum

Tiny ball of wax

That Tiny Ball of Candle Wax

Temporally impaired hearing can result when a tiny ball of cerumen is accidently left in the entrance of the canal by an untrained holistic provider that cannot be dumped out by merely tilting the head to the side and may even be pushed deeper inside the outer ear canal when the ear candle is inserted again. A trained technician must be aware of what's going on at all times, especially when fire is being used in such a unique way.

The tiny ball of wax may be removed by flipping it out with an ear pick, a special tool made in China, or carefully with a Q-tip that has been dipped and squeezed of alcohol.

Using sharp or blunt objects to remove ear wax can penetrate the eardrum and dislocate or fracture the stapes bone. Such an injury can cause severe pain and bleeding. If disequilibria should occur, a staggering gait will hinder walking straight. Emergency medical treatment is needed to correct the damage without a moment's delay.

The tiny, yeast-covered ball of ear wax may be seen without the use of an otoscope, an instrument used for inspecting the interior wall of the outer ear as the light source projects a beam, making details of the ear visible through a magnified lens, when the technician is aware of the possibility of its presence.

However, an otoscope cannot view inside the folds of skin that make up the canal, not even by a medical physician. This is the space wherein candidacies (frothy powdered yeast) and other infectious materials can hide in the darkness of the moist surface. With the opening of the mouth during yawning, this fungus can seep in and hide. This is when the gentle warmth of the smoke penetrates the opening and expels the toxic matter.

That tiny cerumen ball has nowhere to go as it cannot go beyond the eardrum, but its presence may hinder clear reception.

What Happened in Ketchum, Idaho?

In the small town of Ketchum, Idaho, I was informed of a medical doctor who had literally caused ear coning treatments to be banned from the area when too many of its townspeople complained of ear infection and an uncomfortable feeling inside the ear canal. When the source of the problem was uncovered, a tiny ball of cerumen had been left at the opening of the external ear and was unknowingly pushed in by a foreign object. As a result, the ear cone novices lost their credibility to which they could contribute to the use of a poorly engineered ear cone that had been distributed throughout this little community or the lack of training of its proper use.

When the local newspaper blew the whistle, the doctors benefited from the scare and the use of ear cones was discontinued there . . . or was it?

The Most Important Final Step

After the complete treatment is finished, it would be best to place a clean cloth over your mouth and nose, and without shaking the jar in any way, carefully observe the mixture of grossness that has been eliminated.

Avoid inhaling or making physical contact with your eyes. Wash hands with alcohol thereafter. This is dead material that has been in the folds of skin of the outer ear since birth . . . or since the last time only one cone was used in each ear in an improper treatment. (One cone per ear is never sufficient enough to be considered effective.)

It is vital that you clean your hands with an antibacterial solution mixed with alcohol prior to removing your face mask. This will eliminate the intake of invisible toxic fumes and airborne yeast infestation.

Ear candling may not be the healthiest holistic practice if measures are not taken to assure that you don't breathe in someone else's toxicity. However, with caution and cleanliness, you will remain in control of every situation. We've been aware of this factor since beginning this treatment many years ago and have found it to be a safe and efficient way to maintain good health standards.

As an extra safety precaution, always be aware of where the flame is; keeping an eye on it every few seconds will avoid mishaps.

Also, avoid the flame being fueled by a breeze or draft from an open window or door. This is one treatment that should never be performed outside unless in an enclosed area, patio or room.

Proper Cleanup Is Essential!

Wherever you are doing a treatment, at home, at our facilities, or in your own office, proper cleanup is a must due to the nature of the service rendered. You will want to first get rid of the pungent debris by discarding it into a plastic (grocery store) bag with *no holes* in it and seal along with all other waste materials derived from the treatment.

Remove all other waste with a plastic glove and empty dirty water into the commode and flush. Be sure to hold skewer at edge of aluminum bowl so only water can escape. You won't want to be responsible for clogging up anyone's toilet.

To clean aluminum bowl and scissors: Hold bowl (and scissors) carefully with a pot holder over a low flame just long enough (three to four seconds) for excess wax to melt away; rotate bowl (and scissors), immediately wipe clean, and shine with a soft cloth. They will look clean and ready for your next treatment. Always clean equipment for appearance as well as good hygiene.

Discard debris in closed waste receptacle out of doors and out of the reach of children and pets.

The toxic substance has been proven to cause nausea, migraine headaches, and dizziness *if inhaled.* Never leave glass jar open to breath in toxic waste. Parasites (microorganisms) die when exposed to air and will expel an odor similar to that of Naugahyde. Keep away from face and exposed skin and never allow children to play or tamper with it.

Always follow instructions for your protection.

How Much Should Ear Coning Treatment Cost?

The average adult ear candling treatment can range from $100 to $125 per two-hour session using six cones, three per ear.

It is an acceptable gesture to offer a senior citizen's discount of 25 percent from the age of fifty-five. Children between the ages of two and ten may benefit from only two cones—one per ear, especially when there is more than one child in the family. This treatment may cost from $25 to $35 for each child.

An extra cone may be provided to adults (at no extra cost) determined by the amount of excessive wax being extracted when one ear may appear to be more impacted than the other. It is best to offer a good, effective treatment as required to relieve pressure or the feeling of stuffiness than to be overly concerned with charges.

In any event, be prepared to be pampered by your trained ear coneologist in a pleasant and quiet environment as the pleasant sound of "crackling" tickles the tympanic, filtering vibrations of meditative relaxation throughout your entire body. We really don't know of any other noninvasive, holistic treatment that can leave you so calm. Providing sootheing music in the background allows your client to enjoy a couple hours away from the stress that brought him in.

When NOT to Treat Ears Holistically

When there's an obvious problem with excess fluids, pain, injury, or extreme pressure, you may notice the bulging of the eardrum (tympanic membrane) as it may appear to be swollen. This is not a symptom you should try to treat or engage the service of a holistic care provider *under any circumstance*. The patient should immediately consult a medical doctor or an ENT specialist to diagnose the symptoms.

That Strip of Candle Wax

Throughout each sequence of the candling process, you will see a 1"-1½" inch long strip of rolled light brown cone wax, first being tapped from a slightly warm candle, approximately two inches in length that did not come from anyone's ear! This odd-shaped piece of candle wax is covered with yeast when it comes out of the cone itself. That's yours!

Precautious Measure

In order to avoid getting water inside the cone, never allow the cone to get wet in the bowl of waste water. Dripping water could make a client feel uncomfortable or startled.

This powdery substance is removed by pushing the skewer inside the cone, dislodging it. Then tap the entire length of the cone with the skewer after cutting off the burnt and blackened portion of the cloth cone. Pay attention to the estimated fire line on each of the candles.

The Best Quality Ear Cone

Pure Beeswax vs. Paraffin

The best feature about the 100 percent pure beeswax cone is that it is 90 percent drip less and burns smoothly for the required two cuts that are made before discarding the remaining (approximately two inches left on the end.

The Paraffin Candle

This candle burns swiftly and a paper or tin pie pan is usually used to keep the dripping wax from falling onto the head or ear. The disadvantage is that you can't see the smoke when it escapes since the cone is burned down as the contents escapes into the room.

What Is Ear Tinnitus?

When a person experiences such sounds as roaring, hissing, buzzing, ear ringing, tinkling, or thumping in the ear that has become persistent, he may have developed tinnitus.

Tinnitus often results from damage to the nerves in the inner ear that may have been caused by prolonged exposure to loud noise such as that from a blasting radio or boom box. This generation of young men and boys seeking attention, with a need to be noticed, will have a rude awakening when they discover the damage they have caused to the tiny hairs inside the cochlea when their hearing becomes irreversibly damaged.

I recall being at a service station filling my tank when a car pulled in behind me with music blasting. I introduced myself (and my profession) and informed the driver of this fact. All he said was, "yeah, that's what my mother tells me all the time."

Tinnitus may also be caused by excess earwax, fluid in the middle ear, infection, dental problems, head or ear injuries, and drugs prescribed by a medical physician. An over—indulgence in alcohol and caffeine can make existing tinnitus worsen. Rarely does it cause brain tumors. When tinnitus is first localized in one ear, you should immediately see an ENT specialist.

Determined by the medical profession that tinnitus has no cure, an ear candling treatment may prove to be the best solution for immediate relief. You don't have to live with the problem just because the doctor said there is no cure. Ear candling is a last-resort remedy that could save thousands of dollars and hours of needless worry and pain. It is certainly worth giving it your utmost consideration.

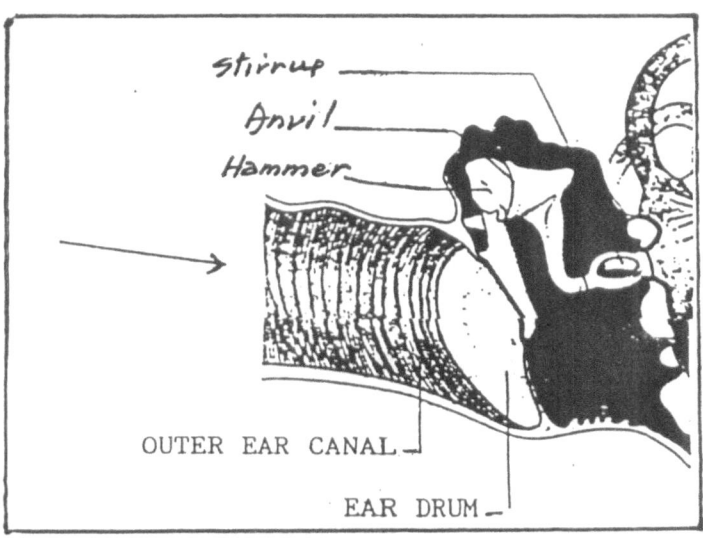

Folds of skin/Outer Ear Canal

Take note of the folds of skin inside the outer ear canal. This area is only 3/4" (20mm) in length and holds as much as two tablespoons of the toxic powdery substance. Candida is a golden color, darker than the cone, or its residue that has been packed inside and is superfluous to the presence of water or oils. They don't mix.

The cool smoke vapor softens the deeply congested matter inside the folds of skin and alleviates ear stress that may cause headaches, deafness, hypertension, and other unnecessary ear maladies such as Bell's palsy. Once Bell's palsy has been treated by a medical doctor, the disease may reoccur since the original problem was not properly treated (holistically) with ear candling.

Chapter IV

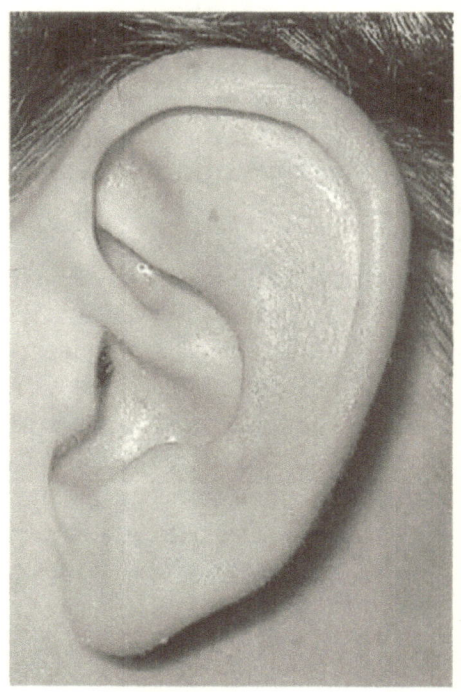

The EXTERNAL EAR

Parts of the Human Ear

involved during the ear coning treatment

The External ear
and
The Outer ear

The External Ear

The exterior part of the ear is where the ear cone is gently placed. It does not have to be deeply inserted as only the smoke need enter the canal in order to work properly. When smoke is escaping, it is not being used properly.

The Outer Ear

The outer ear arrows indicate the direction in which smoke travels osmotically through the ear canal then equalizes concentration during an ear coning treatment.

Parts of the ear not directly involved with
the holistic ear candling procedure include:

The Middle Ear

Location of the ear drum
Hammer/Anvil/Stirrupand Eustachian tube

The Inner Ear

Location of the Cochlea
and Labyrinth

and
The Mastoid Process
(Bone cells)

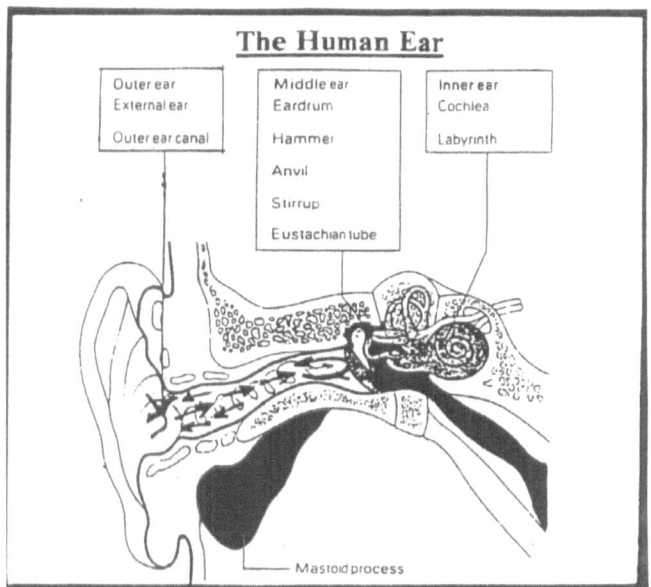

The Mastoid Process

This irregular-shaped process is the mastoid portion of the temporal bone that extends downward and forward behind the external auditory meatus. The air spaces in the mastoid process of the temporal bone are called mastoid cells. Inflammation of these air cells is called mastoiditis.

Diagram Details

Description

A. Middle Ear Infections
B. Myringotomy Procedure
C. Enlarged Outer Ear Canal
D. Frontal Section of the Human Ear

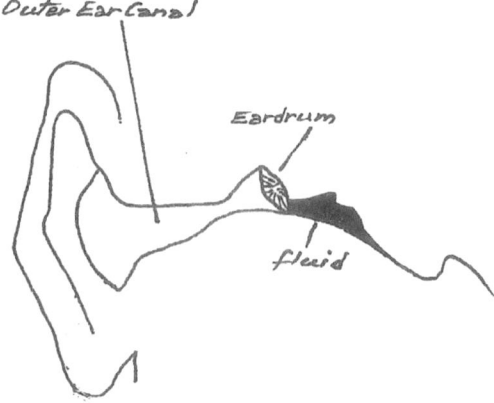

(A) Middle Ear Infection

A. Diagram shows Middle Ear infection.
Fluid is behind the eardrum (Tympanic Membrane)

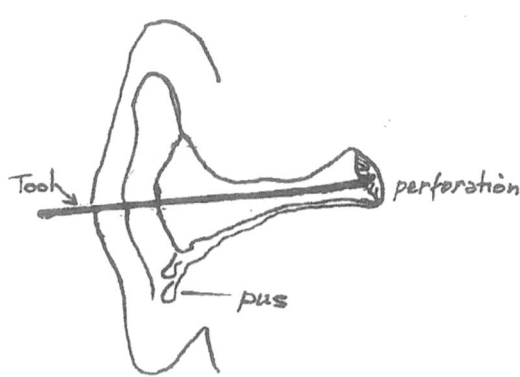

(B) Myringotomy Procedure

B. Diagram shows a myringotomy being done with
instrument that perforates the eardrum.

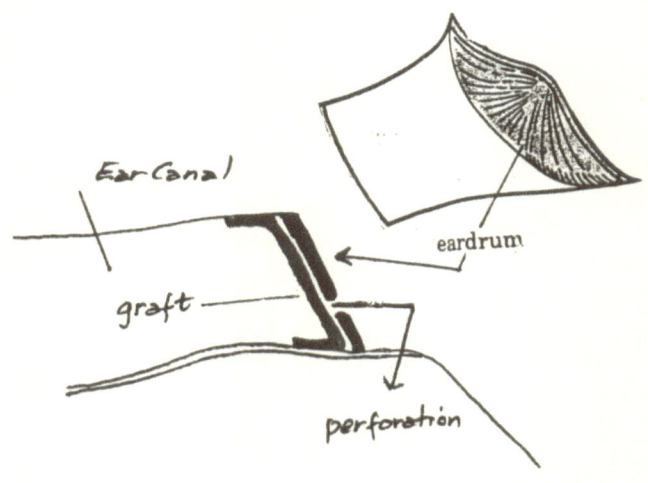

Ear Canal

eardrum

graft

perforation

(C) Enlarged Outer Ear Canal

This diagram shows enlarged outer ear canal and the repairs required on a perforated eardrum. Tissue is grafted from the temporalis muscle on the side of the head to close the perforation. If structures in the inner ear will work freely again, hearing may improve but will never be the same after this procedure.

"Doctor, can we talk?"

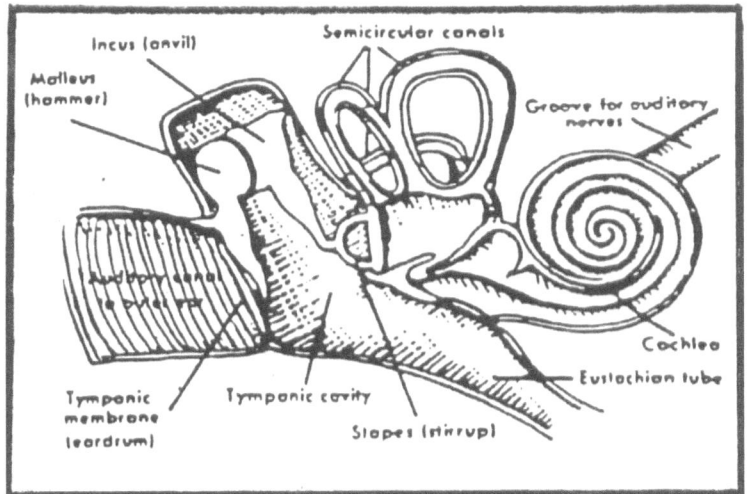

Incus (anvil)

Semicircular canals

Malleus (hammer)

Groove for auditory nerves

Auditory canal

Cochlea

Eustachian tube

Tympanic membrane (eardrum)

Tympanic cavity

Stapes (stirrup)

(D) Frontal Section of the Human Ear

This diagram shows the folds of skin located inside the auditory canal of the outer ear where yeast and other parasites, fungi, debris, and virus thrive in the moist dark crevices.

Chapter V

Our First Grads—July 2000

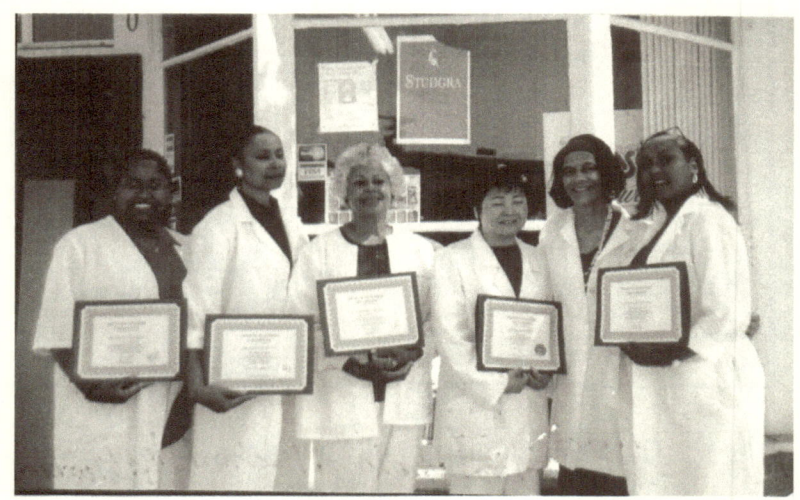

**Introduction to
THE SYLLABUS
Basic Approach to the
Ancient Art of Ear Candling**

**Institute of Certified Ear Candler's
QUESTIONS and ANSWERS**

The QUESTIONS

Suggestion:

Read each question first to get familiar with it.

The External Ear

1. What are the three major parts of the external ear?
2. What is the primary purpose of the ear?

The Outer Ear

1. What best describes the outer ear?
2. How long is the passage that leads from the pinna to the tympanic membrane?
3. What covers the pinna, and what purpose does it serve?
4. How is the deeper part of the ear canal constructed?
5. What is another name for the tympanic membrane?
6. What purpose does the tympanic membrane serve?
7. What does the structure of the ear do, and what is its primary purpose?

The Middle Ear

1. What is the middle ear, and where is it located?
2. What three small bones connect with the middle ear?
3. What is attached to the inner lining of the eardrum?
4. What is attached by a ligament to the oval window?
5. What is the oval window?

6. What is the purpose of the stirrup or stapes bone?
7. What is attached to both the hammer and the stirrup?
8. What are the three openings of the middle ear?
9. What is the temporal bone, and what is it used for?
10. What is the Eustachian tube?
11. What is the auditory canal?
12. What happens when the auditory tube is blocked as when one suffers from sinus congestion or viral infection?

The Inner Ear

1. What are the two membrane-lined structures of the inner ear?
2. What are they filled with?
3. What is the labyrinth?
4. What is the cochlea?
5. Where does hearing start?
6. What connects hearing and balance functions?
7. What are the two main functions of the inner ear?
8. What is vertigo?
9. What is the major symptom of vertigo?
10. What is the main function of the inner ear?

Infections of the Outer Ear Canal

1. What is the medical term for ear disorders?
2. What are two forms of ear infection?
3. What causes otitis-externa?

Hearing Loss

1. What are two kinds of major hearing loss causes?
2. What is conductive hearing loss?
3. What causes conductive loss of hearing?
4. What is sensorineural loss?
5. What causes this disorder of hearing loss?
6. What is the major cause of ear problems and damage caused to the auditory canal nerve endings?
7. What are four other causes of ear loss damage?

Description of the ICEC Distant Learning Course

Chapter I
Read book and review before beginning test

Chapter II
Basic Approach to the Ancient Art of Ear Candling

Chapter III
Completion
Ten Hours Externship and Performance
Final Written Test (Open Book Q&A)
Your Hands-On Demonstration
This is your performance in a ten minute video or
(6) recent photographs (8 1/2 X 11) or 5X6 of you performing a
treatment. Verification of (5) clients served by you
prior to receiving your beautiful certificate of completion.

Your dress code picture is requested for the school year book.
Uniform: White shirt/white shoes and socks/white smock
Option: ICEC logo on back and name on left shirt pocket
$85 for embroidery on your smock

Chapter IV
Know Your Tools of the Trade
(Please list minimum of 15 required items)

BEST QUALITY EAR CONES

Our cones are hand-made especially for the
Institute of Certified Ear Candler's

Sold in six-pack for one full treatment
$36

Sold in two-pack for emergency treatment
$15

One dozen ear cones at $75
For two full treatments at six cones per ear

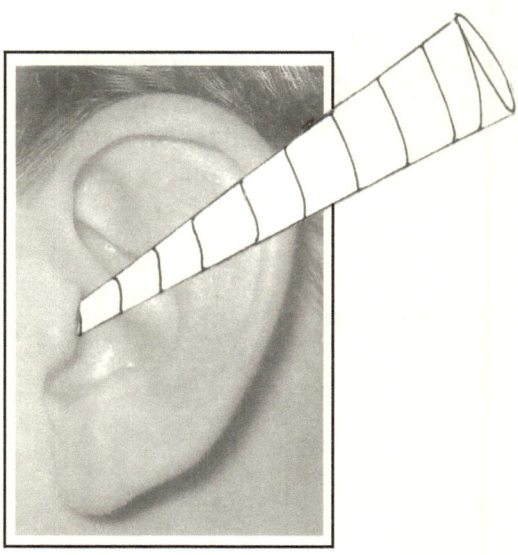

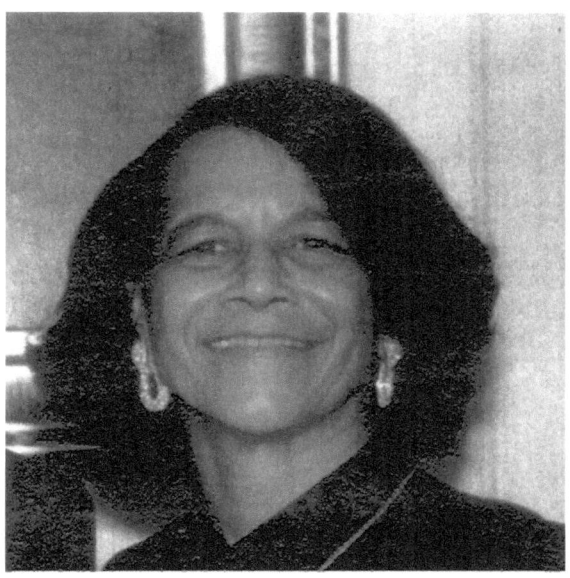

Penny Rich

About the Author

Penny Rich is a state-certified/registered ear coneologist, holistic practitioner, and clinical hypnotherapist as a graduate of the Hypnosis Motivation Institute (HMI) in Tarzana, California, in 1990.

Self-hypnosis and clinical hypnotherapy deal with matters of the mind not resolved through the medical profession, in order to produce dynamic results that create effective and beneficial changes in mental dexterity, skills, techniques, and verbal tools required to more effectively handle personal relationships and life's experiences. Hypnosis develops the communication skills needed to enhance the inner wisdom and guidance that determines the cause and affect solutions to issues we may find perplexing throughout life that began within the formative years of our growth, only to manifest throughout our adult years.

Penny is a thirteen-year veteran of cable television, having written and produced *The Penny Rich Show,* which aired from the Los Angeles studio of the formerly owned Continental Cablevision, to Media One, to Comcast, and now owned by Time Warner, concurrently writing and producing her own radio show on KTYM-FM, Inglewood, California, from 1985 to the turn of the century, 2003.

Quite a legacy was left by those who were so dedicated to the advancement of television production on cable televisions. It was during the 80s when all you had to do was show up on time to put your show on . . . or be fined $20 for having their production crew waiting for you to take your dream to be in television more seriously. It was public television at a premium, operated by a few of those same folks who were just students themselves then, students who would eventually wind up on one of the *real* television productions networks where they may still be . . . thirty years later . . .

Penny wrote and produced a sixty-second spot for her radio commercial, "Have You Learned How to Manage Money Yet?" featuring her numerology business as a master numerologist with her own dedicated (900 Line). However, it aired on the Wave/FM radio station six weeks prior to the Northridge earthquake in California that occurred on January 17, 1994, at 4:31 a.m. when it struck the San Fernando Valley causing a lack of interest in the subject.

She became a Master Numerologist in 1985. Through the science of numbers comes the release of the "crutch" that represents ones shortcomings as karmic obligations that she presents in an amazingly accurate countdown of your destiny through experiences that are recognized in your given name and date of birth. This is profoundly incredible information that can keep track of who you are and basically how your life is to go as a mortal being of the realm, or perhaps even as an earthbound archangel in human flesh.

Penny's book, *Archangel of the Earth Realm—Entertained Unawares* is a non-fiction, compeling story relating to the experiences entrusted to an earthbound archangel living her life as a mortal being commissioned to serve mankind

Her book, *Children Owe Karma Too!* details the karmic obligations related to children of all ages as a guide to raising children utilizing the nine karmic clues found in numeric evaluations.

From 1985 to 1995, she wrote a weekly newspaper column "Rich Wisdom" featuring her story-poetry on the drama of daily dilemmas for a local tabloid, *Scoop News*. Her thirty-six-verse poem, "My Name Is Crack and I'm Talkin' Back," began a ten-year internship as a newspaper columnist.

In 1972, Penny graduated from the Chicago School of Interior Decoration, a home study course which led to a thirty-seven-year career as an independent commercial/residential interior decorator specializing in wallpaper sales and service. Penny gained respect and recognition as "The Lady Wallpaper Hanger" throughout Southern California until she retired in 2007 to launch her writing career.

In 1990, the Institute of Certified Ear Candler's was founded. Penny is also co-founder and Director of Admissions.

Now that she has perused almost every venue of journalism and communication, the time finally came when writing would fulfill her passion for creative expression as an author.

The ANSWERS

(All answers must be in complete sentences.

These answers are for the QUESTIONS they relate to. Incomplete answers receive a five-point reduction [each] off score and may cause failure of the test.)

Remember, the answers are well defined throughout the text. However, if you would like to research the answers on the Web, feel free to increase your understanding, knowledge, and enhance your final score. Good luck!

1. External ear has three major parts:
   (A) The outer (pinna) external ear perceives sound.
   (B) The middle ear has five parts located in auditory canal.
       (1) Tympanic, eardrum, thin membrane separates middle ear from the external ear and vibrates when struck by sound waves.
       (2) Hammer, or malleus, one of the bones located in the middle ear.
       (3) Anvil means to beat.
       (4) Stirrup or stapes means to support.
       (5) The Eustachian tube, a slender tube between the middle ear and the pharynx, which serves to equalize air pressure on both sides of eardrums.
           The Anatomist who dissected and analyzed the ear was Bartolommeo Eustachio for which the Eustachian tube was named. (1520—1574).

(C) The inner ear is the farthest inside. It has two parts: cochlea, meaning snail, a spiral-shaped part of the inner ear containing auditory nerve endings, and the labyrinth, meaning intricate winding structure.

2. Purpose: Dedicated to hearing and balance (equilibrium).

The outer ear:
1. Description: Includes parts of ear we can see. Inside are visible folds of skin and cartilage. Small bones and cartilage consist of a gristly skeleton.
2. Length of passage from pinna to eardrum is only ¾" long and 20mm in folds of skin layers.
3. This cartilage is covered with tiny hairs that filter dust and protect wax-producing glands.
4. It is lined by a thin membrane surrounded by bone and cartilage.
5. The tympanic membrane—a thin percussive layer of skin that stretches across the end of the outer ear canal.
6. Eardrum separates sound waves and funnels them into middle ear, then passes them into the inner ear.
7. It collects sound waves and funnels them into middle ear, then passes them on to the inner ear.

The middle ear:
1. Small cavity located between eardrum and inner ear.
2. Three small bones: the hammer, the anvil, and the stirrup or stapes.
3. The hammer is attached to inner lining of eardrum.
4. The oval window has two membrane-covered openings or outlets into which the air-filled middle ear of the oval window and the round window vibrates with opposite phase of motion.
5. A membrane-covered opening leads from middle ear to vestibule of inner ear.
6. Purpose of stirrups: To transmit movement to oval window. As stapes footplate moves into oval window, the round window membrane moves out, and this allows movement of fluids within cochlea, leading to movement of cochlea's inner tiny hair cells, and thus, hearing occurs.

7. The anvil is attached to hammer and stirrup.
8. There are three openings in middle ear. One leads to air spaces located in mastoid region or near a projection of the temporal bone behind ear known as the mastoid projection. Two other openings lead to the inner ear.
9. Temporal bone contains all internal regions of ear, located near the temple on the flat surface behind the forehead and to the front of the ear. It is either of a pair of compound bones forming the sides of the skull.
10. Eustachian tube is the passage between pharynx and inner ear that forms auditory canal, the eardrum cavity of the middle ear, and pinna (external) ear.
11. Auditory canal is the passage between pharynx and inner ear that forms auditory canal and serves to equalize air pressure between inner ear, the eardrum cavity of middle and external ear.
12. Sudden equalization causes ears to pop. Unequal pressure can be very painful and annoying. Removal of yeast and other parasites and toxic waste is the most effective treatment in relieving unnecessary ear maladies, accomplished through ear candling.

The inner ear:
1. Has two membrane-covered outlets leading into the air-filled middle ear—the cochlea and the labyrinth.
2. Fluids.
3. A semicircular canal consisting of three connected tubes bent into half circles located in the middle ear.
4. Part of the inner ear dedicated to the ability of hearing.
5. Hearing starts in inner side of oval window, shaped like an egg and curls around like a snail.
6. Connect hearing with balance attaching themselves to the labyrinth and cochlea.
7. Contains mechanism for maintaining good balance of equilibrium; converts sound waves into nerve impulses that are then transmitted to the brain.
8. An ear disorder. Vertigo gives a false sense of the room spinning.
9. May cause loss of balance, dizziness.
10. Senses movement and maintains good balance when not infested with excess wax and natural debris.

Infections of the outer ear canal:
1. Otitis-externa.
2. Generalized: Disorders that affect the entire ear lining.
   Localized: Boils, abscesses such as yellow-green pus infections that often occur to very young children.
3. Swimming in polluted water.
   Persistent and excessive moisture in ear canal.
   Scratching inside ear to relieve or remove hardened ear wax.
   Itching followed by an annoying pain.
   When pus seeps out, pain is often relieved; but when it dries, it may cause serious blockage in ear canal.
   The best way to avoid disorders is to treat your ears to a one-hour relaxing ear candling treatment performed by a qualified and trained tech.

Hearing Loss:
1. Conductive and sensorineural.
2. Conductive hearing loss is a mechanical failure that prevents sound from reaching the inner ear.
3. Caused by wax blockage in inner ear.
4. When one or more of the 4,000+ nerve endings suffers a failure to communicate. Sound that does reach the inner ear is not passed on to the brain for clarity.
5. Candida (yeast infestation), a golden substance that clogs the ear canal with bits of hardened ear wax, parasites, and other normal debris.
6. Sensorineural hearing loss caused when there is damage to the cochlea or auditory nerve endings.
7. Four causes for ear damage and hearing loss:
   a. Loud music machinery
   b. Excessive pounding and drum beats from loud music and car radio vibrations.
   c. Rare side effects from medications
   d. Gunfire, explosives, and especially firecrackers
   (E) All of the above.

<End of test>

Tools of the Trade

A warm and cordial personality
A professional appearance and rapport
Patience and watchful concern

Aluminum quart-sized bowl
Medium-sized sharp scissors (with extra pair)
Small glass (jelly) jar with lid (approx. three inches) for debris
Plastic (grocery store) waste bags
100% Cotton balls
Alcohol or raw vinegar
Lighter (without safety catch)
Wax candle for lighting cone
Towels (for shoulders and head wrap)
Two small pillows for head and between knees
Face mask
Plastic gloves for handling debris
Two dozen best quality cones for four sessions

One massage table
One fold-up chair with back support
One fold-up small side table

Your ear candling kit on wheels is available with everything you will need to get started. It includes two dozen all-natural, unscented best quality ear cones.
For $85 (includes shp/hndl)

Important Tips Re: Cleanup Process

- Always empty dirty water from aluminum bowl into toilet, and be sure to hold stick over lip of bowl to prevent debris from falling into toilet. Never flush toilet with burnt candle debris, cone wax, and candling debris that has fallen in—that you must remove with gloved hand. Inform and/or show client your method to prevent this from happening or you will be held responsible for an expensive plumbing bill.

- Remove trash from bowl and place into plastic bowl for disposal outside in covered trash container.

- Clean hands with alcohol or raw vinegar.

The Ear Candler's Disclaimer Form

The ear coning process is not to be considered a medical treatment, and no such claim is being made as such. It is an ancient, holistic ear cone vapor bath that has found its way into the twenty-first century as a safe, beneficial, and practical holistic remedy for the maintenance and well-being of the outer ear canal.

Those participating in ear candling (or coning) must assume full responsibility for its use and may not hold anyone liable—not the manufacturer, the seller, or the certified practitioner who performs the non-invasive procedure on self or others. It is, however, highly recommended that a trained technician perform the treatment and that it not be done without the watchful eyes of a second party.

We shall not be held responsible for any claims, expenses incurred, or any damages caused by careless incident.

In the years we have performed the ear candling treatment, neither ICEC nor any of our students have ever experienced adverse occurrence.

Those being treated acknowledge that they have read, understood, and signed a similar disclaimer form at the time of treatment and recognize the importance of medical advice and treatment in the resolve of any medical-related ear malady.

Penny Rich, CEC
Certified Ear Candler
and Holistic Practitioner

Other Mind-Body-Spirit Books

By Penny Rich

- New:
  Archangel of the Earth Realm—Entertained Unawares

- Self-Help—Numerology
  Children Owe Karma Too!
  Nine Karmic Clues to Raising Children